How to Im Memory & Increase Your Brain Power in 30 Days

Simple, Easy & Fun Ways to Improve Memory Now

By: Jason Scotts

TABLE OF CONTENTS

PUBLISHERS NOTES

Disclaimer

This publication is intended to provide helpful and informative material. It is not intended to diagnose, treat, cure, or prevent any health problem or condition, nor is intended to replace the advice of a physician. No action should be taken solely on the contents of this book. Always consult your physician or qualified health-care professional on any matters regarding your health and before adopting any suggestions in this book or drawing inferences from it.

The author and publisher specifically disclaim all responsibility for any liability, loss or risk, personal or otherwise, which is incurred as a consequence, directly or indirectly, from the use or application of any contents of this book.

Any and all product names referenced within this book are the trademarks of their respective owners. None of these owners have sponsored, authorized, endorsed, or approved this book.

Always read all information provided by the manufacturers' product labels before using their products. The author and publisher are not responsible for claims made by manufacturers.

© 2013

Manufactured in the United States of America

DEDICATION

This book is dedicated to my family whose unyielding support gave me the drive to get things done no matter how difficult the process may be.

CHAPTER 1- MEMORY- WHAT IS IT AND WHY IS IT SO IMPORTANT?

There are a variety of definitions for memory; let's look at the most common meanings.

Memory is defined as "the ability to store and retain information from daily experiences; archive this information in folders for use at a later date."

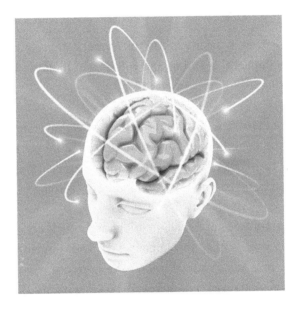

There are different types of memory our brain can store, they are:

1. Short term

2. Long term

3. Sensory

4. Explicit

5. Implicit

6. Episodic

7. Semantic

Your short term memory, also known as "working memory," is the type of memory we use most often. This part of our memory bank is used for daily functions such as calculations, writing letters, conversations, and onetime events. The impact a particular experience has on us also determines how long we remember things.

If you're involved in a car accident or robbery; these are situations that greatly impact the victims and will stick in their memories for a very long time.

Recall - when talking about what memory is, we must include recall as part of the definition. It's one thing to retain information and it is another to extract it from the memory banks. This two part process is what makes memory a vital part of learning.

Sensory Memory - sight, smell, hearing, and touch are all forms of sensory memory. Again, the impact each experience has on you determines how long you will retain the memory. For example, if you went to a restaurant and had a really fantastic meal, this would have a positive impact on you that could last for a long time. The opposite could also be true, and in this case your recall mechanism kicks in reminding you of restaurants you don't want to revisit again.

Why is Your Memory Important?

Memory and Learning - this is one of the main reasons memory is so important. Imagine having to ask the same question over and over again because you cannot remember the answer. There wouldn't be the progress and development in technology we see today. Everything we do is based on memory. You have to remember how to get home from work. Do you remember how to get to your friends house? How about the wedding anniversary? Forgetting this can cause a lot of tension in your life.

Memory and Making a Living - people don't connect the two - memory and work. You must depend on your memory, both short and long term, to perform daily functions. Yes, you can write things down in lieu of having to remember them but imagine the time it would take to do daily tasks. If anything, you should be increasing your memory capacity and reducing your dependency on lists for routine jobs.

Pain and Pleasure - memory is important so we can avoid those things causing us pain and continue with those things that give us pleasure. One of the best examples is in the food category. Everybody likes to eat sweets, but not everyone can process the glucose properly and the end result is a big, fat headache. So when the next urge for sweets hits, hopefully the memory of the pain that follows will deter that person from indulging. The reality is - even with the memory of pain, the urge sometimes still wins.

Memory and Skills - this type of memory is in conjunction with learning, but it is more specific to a skill. One of the best examples is sports. Playing basketball requires a lot of hours of practice, practicing plays and repetitive shooting exercises. The purpose of practicing shots hundreds, if not thousands of times, is to build a reactive memory. In a game situation the player doesn't have time to think about the shot, they just have to react. This is the whole purpose of practicing - building a memory to master a particular skill.

This type of memory applies to most sports such as golf, tennis, baseball, soccer, and hockey.

Memory and Survival - this type of memory is right up there with learning except we're talking about "loss of memory." It is vital for our survival to remember to do things. Believe it or not, some people forget to eat and become nutritionally starved. There are too many stories of people who forget to turn off the stove and burn down their house - sometimes the results can even be more fatal. The medical terms for this type of degenerative memory loss is referred to as "Dementia and Alzheimer's."

Exercising Your Memory

Keeping your memory in shape is just as important as keeping your body fit. There are memory techniques you can use such as "pegging," and there are games you can play to exercise your brain like "pairs."

In a world where we have calculators, computers that spell check, and electronic gadgets that keep track of everything we don't want to remember, we are relinquishing our capacity of memory. As you have read, you use your memory in every aspect of your life. Have you heard the old saying "if you don't use it you will lose it?" Well, this also applies to your memory.

This is why it's important to exercise and expand the capacity of your memory and not let modern conveniences replace the need for memory. People have been mislead into thinking that memory loss is a natural digression, but we know of people in their 90's that are just as sharp as they were 30 years ago. What's the secret? Well, there are three things we see they have in common - they are:

1. Reading

2. Puzzles (crossword)

3. Nutrition

These elders read a lot, they do puzzles daily, and they are very particular about their diet. They didn't just start doing these things when they hit ninety; they incorporated these habits into their lifestyles many years earlier.

Your memory is vitally important for survival and quality of life. If you do some of the simple things to keep it fit now, your memory will serve you well throughout your lifetime.

CHAPTER 2- THE ADVANTAGES OF BOOSTING MEMORY

It is important to have a strong memory since it is important to your health and your brain's vitality. Whether you are a high school or college student who is studying for finals, a working person who is concerned about maintaining mental sharpness, or an elderly person who is searching for ways to preserve their gray matter in the aging process, you can improve your mental performance along with keeping your memory sharp.

You may wonder why your memory is so important. Your memory can be thought of as a filing system for your brain. It stores every single thing that you have learned throughout your lifetime. The brain can actually store a huge amount of information. When you were young, you learned about ten words a day that were new to you. As an adult, you probably know more than 100,000 words.

Your brain consists of 100 billion neurons. As you get older, these neurons are wired together and they communicate through tons of connections called synapses. When some of these connections are made stronger, memories are formed. Therefore, boosting your memory is important to prevent the aging process from destroying the memories you have formed over the years.

Believe it or not, spending time with friends is a great memory booster. Many people think of serious and tough activities when they think of improving their memory. However, this is not the case all the time. Improving your sharpness is not all about crossword puzzles or playing chess. Hanging out with friends and laughing while having fun has cognitive benefits.

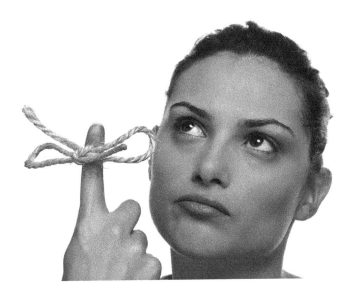

As human beings, we are very social and we cannot survive alone. We also cannot thrive when we are alone all the time. Therefore, this is why it is important to form healthy relationships in order to stimulate your brain activity. In fact, studies have shown that being with people you like to be around is the best form of brain exercise. You can begin to take advantage of socializing by doing things like volunteering, joining a club or making plans to visit friends more often.

Supplements are another way to increase your memory power. With alarming statistics like 10 million baby boomers suffering from Alzheimer's disease, the elderly population is always looking for ways to enhance their memory. However, do supplements really work for this purpose? It seems that herbal supplements are recommended more than prescription medications. The problem with prescription medication is that they are very costly and they sometimes have limited effectiveness in a short time window.

Experts have discovered that there are certain foods that increase your memory. The Alzheimer's Association calls these brain-healthy foods. These foods are said to lessen the chance of getting heart disease and diabetes and encourages increased blood flow to your brain. These foods include blackberries, apples, cinnamon, spinach, chocolate, and salmon. They are all rich in DHEA, or good fats that feed the brain.

Ginkgo Biloba is the most common and most popular supplement used for enhancing memory. It is commonly used in Europe to treat a form of dementia that occurs from lack of blood flow. By taking Ginkgo Biloba, it helps to improve blood flow in small blood vessels. Other supplements such as Huperzine A, Vitamin E, and Omega-3 fatty acids have all been shown to improve memory.

There are several advantages to boosting your memory.

Boosting memory defines who we are. If you suddenly lost all of your memories, you would not have any sense of who you are. It is the experiences that you have had in your past that will determine who and what will allow in your future. After all, with no memory of your past, you really cannot move forward to your future. We need to form and build relationships so we are able to define whom we are.

Improving your memory helps you learn and to prosper. Your memory is important because it is what helps you learn new things as well as foster new skills. It was proven that to be important in school, we needed to memorize several various pieces of information, so that we could pass certain classes such as math and history. We heavily rely on our memory to study for tests and to learn recitations. These skills are used later in life in the professions that we choose. You do not want a nurse working on you in the hospital that cannot remember how to do basic math to give you the appropriate increase of medication.

Memory is a huge part of your working atmosphere. While it is true that you do not have to take tests most of the time when you are employed, your memory is still needed to remember meetings you

Jason Scotts

have and schedules you need to adhere to. No matter what your occupation is, you need your memory to perform your job duties efficiently. If you fail to do things in the appropriate order, or constantly need supervision for assistance, you could lose your job.

When you build relationships with others, you will need your memory to help you remember people's names when you first meet them. Having a great memory also helps you to remember people's birthdays and anniversaries. While this may not seem important to some, others know that people care about them when important things to them are remembers. For example, remembering the names of someone's children shows that you care about their life. Taking that further, knowing their children's birthdays, or favorite dinner, or sports they play, will them that you invest in their lives.

Remember, memory is a reflection of your mental process. It does not only define who you are presently, but it also helps ward off mental problems later in life. Many believe, and research is beginning to show, that when you constantly boost your memory, your risk of Alzheimer's, and other dementia disorders goes down significantly. When you have a good memory, it means that you have great brain power. Therefore, when you do what you can to boost your memory, what you are really doing is improving the way that you think.

CHAPTER 3- THE TOP TEN WAYS TO IMPROVE LONG TERM MEMORY

You can help to strengthen your long term memory in many ways. Like a muscle, your memory can be trained through daily exercises and habits. By following these tips, you will be able to constantly improve your long-term memory.

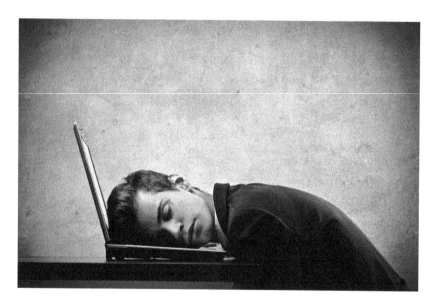

Read and Analyze Literature

Reading classic literature can help to improve your long term memory in many ways. Reading and absorbing masterful prose will allow you to form new thoughts, gain a larger vocabulary, and think more lucidly. Also, keeping track of the many characters and themes will help to keep your mind active.

As you read more, try to expand into different genres and areas of literature. This will keep things fresh and interesting. Having your mind analyze different forms and styles of literature will allow you to form a comprehensive working memory. This will greatly help

Jason Scotts

your long term memory as you compare current texts to ones you have previously read.

Learn a New Language

Learning a language will greatly benefit your long term memory. You will start to see your first language in new ways, and you will keep your mind busy with new grammar and vocabulary. Don't worry; it is never too late to start learning a new language!

You should first learn the basic grammar of your new language. This will be the foundation that you can the build upon as you progress. After you have a basic grasp of the grammar, start to learn key phrases and vocabulary. Use flashcards to get the terms imprinted in your brain. Recalling words is a great form of mental exercise, and your long term memory will thank you for it.

Practice with Puzzles

Puzzles can help to keep your mind sharp and your memory working. Crossword puzzles can help you to recall words you may have forgotten. They will also force you to look up new words in the dictionary which is a great way to learn.

Sudoku is a mathematical puzzle that is also great for the mind. Your mind will grow stronger with each new challenge, and your long term memory will sharpen with the practice. There are many books available for different skill levels, so you can find the right book for you and upgrade when necessary.

Supplementation for Long Term Memory

Even if you do everything right, there are many benefits to be had from supplementation. Adding fish oil is a great way to increase you long term memory. Studies have shown that omega fatty acids are perfect for brain health and cognition. They have shown to slow down the onset of Alzheimer's as well as other degenerative diseases.

There are also many nootropics available to help aid your long term memory. A nootropic is a supplement that carries virtually no risk. The most famous nootropic is Piracetam. Piracetam is reported to help aid visual recall and the formation of new memories. If you wish to regain or increase your long term memory, then Piracetam may help you.

If you are suffering from brain fog, then apple cider vinegar may help. Apple cider vinegar works by cleaning out the system and aiding digestion. Your body will feel cleaner and you will gain more nutrients from your foods. Many people report a feeling of clarity after drinking just a few teaspoons a day. Try using apple cider vinegar to feel more alert and ready to learn new things.

A Proper Diet

A proper diet can help you to feel your best at all times. If you are not receiving all of the proper nutrients you need throughout the day, then you are apt to feel sluggish and mentally tired. You should be eating enough fruits and green vegetables throughout the day, along with a proper protein intake in order to feel your best.

Your long term memory is formed each day, so providing your body with the proper nutrients ensures that your memory is cohesive. You cannot train your mind if your body is low on fuel, so make sure to drink enough water to replenish yourself throughout the day. Avoiding junk food and drinking enough water will help you to advance your long term memory.

Teach Others In Order to Improve Long Term Memory

Teaching others concepts that you understand can greatly help to cement memories for the long term. It allows you to truly understand all aspects of the area you are teaching. Pupils may ask questions from angles you had never imagined. By expressing the answers and solutions in an understandable way, you will further improve your long term memory and understanding.

Physical Exercise Helps to Stimulate Your Mind

Physical exercise helps to keep both your mind and body in shape. Don't neglect your body during your academic pursuits. Training your body allows your mind to perform at an optimal level.

You don't have to be a bodybuilder or marathon runner in order to keep your mind happy, but you do need to put in the work. Do some pushups throughout the day to keep the blood pumping. Go for a walk when your mind is feeling tired. You can also do a quick set of squats in your room in order to release powerful hormones. Even a small amount of exercise each day will greatly help you in keeping your mind healthy and sharp.

Get Enough Sleep

Memories cement themselves into your mind while you're asleep. Make sure to sleep enough each night in order to ensure that your memories are properly developed. A failure to do so will leave you too tired to study and too worn out to remember.

Use Your Senses

Use your senses to help form long term memories. Imagine a visual to correspond with a fact you wish to remember. You can also utilize sounds, scents, and even touch if you're creative. Use whatever works best for you to help keep those memories stored permanently.

Don't Give Up!

Your long term memory always needs to be worked on in order to thrive. Don't get lazy and neglect proper habits. Keep working on it and you will reap the benefits.

CHAPTER 4- THE BEST TECHNIQUES TO IMPROVE MEMORY

There are two ways to improve memory - through nutrition and exercise. This chapter will focus more on exercising your memory muscles for improved memory.

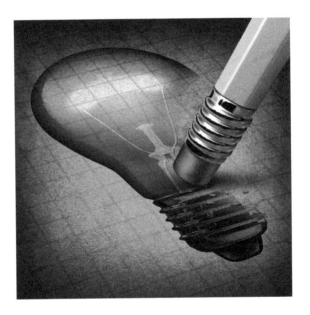

The Link Technique

The link technique is one of the more basic memory methods, but still highly effective.

This technique requires you to create an image you can associate with the item you want to remember. Let's take the names Paul, Bob, and Stan. This is how the linking technique works:

- Paul came over to fix Bobs' car.

- Bob called Stan to see if he could help.

This is a very simple example, but you get the idea. The key to getting the most benefit from this technique is "vivid associations." This means linking to things familiar to you.

Making the images vivid makes the whole pattern more memorable, and you'll be amazed at how easy it becomes to remember list containing 15 or 20 items.

The Story Technique

This technique is a kin to the link method with the exception to structure. The sequencing of the story is ultra important for this method to work.

Let's use the same names - Paul, Bob, and Stan.

Example: I called Paul to see if he wanted to go fishing. Bob said he could go this coming Saturday and he would check with Stan to see if he could make it too.

As you can see, in this example the person has a passion for fishing. Your memory becomes more vivid and stimulated when you use a subject that you're passionate about. The hardest part of this technique is remembering the sequence of the story; as you add more things to your list.

The Alphabet Technique

This alphabet technique is in a group called "the peg system." This method is good for remembering longer lists by associating letters, images, and list.

For this example let's say you need to remember 15 things. You would start by using the first 15 letters of the alphabet - A through O. Lets also say we are remembering a grocery list.

1. A - Apple

2. B - Bee - Honey

3. C - See - Eye Drops

4. D - Dishes - Dish soap

5. E - Electricity - Light bulbs

6. F - Fishing - Salmon for dinner

The key to mastering this memory technique is to relate a meaningful image to each letter. The letter is used to maintain an orderly and memorable sequence, the related image has to be strong so it can relate to the list.

This form of pegging may seem cumbersome at first but science has proven that our brain has a much better capacity for remembering through association.

The Journey Technique

As you might have already guessed, the journey technique is a method by which you peg the item you are trying to remember to specific stops on a journey.

This method is good for remembering lists of information that are non-related. As with all of these techniques, you must spend time learning them to actually master them. Let's use our grocery list to show how this technique works.

The simple journey associated with shopping is going to the market itself.

1. Getting up, turning on the stove: Coffee

2. Showering: Soap

3. Spill orange juice: Paper towels

4. Turn radio on in car: Beets

5. Hit garbage can backing out of driveway: Trash bags

Do you see how the mind works in these situations? We must repeat this again - they journey has to be your journey, something you can associate with. If your routine for going to the market is different from the one above, then make the journey fit what will be memorable to you!

Memory Exercises

Besides learning memory techniques, you can exercise your mind using mind games.

One of the more popular mind exercise games is called "paxeso." You may have also seen this referred to as "pairs." You can use an ordinary deck of playing cards and to start, all you need to do is pair up the cards. Each number or face card will have four cards matched - all you need is two from each group. There should be 13 groups that total 26 cards.

Now, place the 26 cards face down and shuffle them around on the table. Make sure you mix them well and then spread the cards out so they are not clumped on top of each other. Now the fun begins.

Turn one card over, look at it, remember it, and place it face down. You have already guessed what comes next - repeat the step. As you turn over the other cards you will have to remember where the matching cards are and pair them up. The object is to match up all 13 pairs of cards.

Jason Scotts

You'll be able to monitor your progress in two ways; the first is by increasing the cards. By this we mean adding the third card to the exercise. Remember, there are four cards to each number or face card in the deck. Then you'll want to start timing your progress. Time yourself each time you play, log your time and see how you improve.

Online Games - you will be surprised at how many free online brain games are available for you to train with. There are math, I.Q. test, memory tests, reflex tests, and concentration games that will help exercise your memory cells. Just do a simple search for "memory games" and you'll find a bunch of great sites.

The techniques we've outlined here to improve memory are some of the best techniques on the market. These techniques take time to learn and take even more time to master. We suggest learning the ones that will benefit your situation the best. Some of the "peg systems" are complex and may be of no use to you, so why spend the time when the simple "link technique" will work just fine.

We're sure you will find value in learning some of these memory techniques, and you can never go wrong in exercising the most important muscle of all - your brain.

CHAPTER 5- WHY REPETITION IS IMPORTANT FOR MEMORY IMPROVEMENT

Repetition is a necessary building block for long-term memory. Without long-term memory, it would not be possible to interact with other people, make any type of decisions or solve problems. Because life situations are constantly evolving, interactions with people, decisions and problem solving are constantly adjusting and requiring new information to add to the existing.

It is imperative to continue efforts to improve memory and learning throughout one's life in order to function, contribute and enjoy. Although the adult brain has mastered many skills and has massive amounts of information, the adult brain cannot acquire new long term memory or skills without the exercise of repetition. Unless a person is regularly studying and learning, repetitive activities would be necessary to use and enjoy existing knowledge.

Learning by repetition is also known as rote learning. Rote learning has often been criticized because it is very mechanical and does not require understanding. Rote learning is not responsive to questions and curiosity, it is just drill. While learning by repetition, the joy of discovery is missing and learning by repetition often becomes boring and tedious. All of us remember the ABC song or times tables recited to music. Using music and rhythm will make repetition and drill more enjoyable and can help learning.

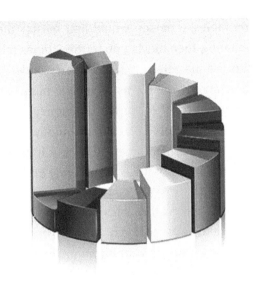

To have learned any information, the information must be converted or stored to long term memory and information will only be learned or stored if it is remembered which requires repetition in the beginning. Mastery of the multiplication tables and the alphabet are good examples of rote learning, or learning by repetition. Even with calculators and computers, lack of mastery of multiplication tables makes mathematical challenges more difficult throughout life. For all people, repetition is necessary in order to remember information, some fortunate people may require only one or two repetitions in order to remember, most people need 6 to 9 repetitions.

To have memory means that a person has received, kept and been able to retrieve or remember any information. Encoding is a term for receiving information by the brain. There are different ways to encode different types of memory that are important. Visual encoding would be similar to storing pictures in the brain.

Elaborative encoding means that information is added to information that is already stored in the brain. For example, in multiplication tables, a person would first master the 1 time, and then the two times, then moving on to the 5 times tables. Once the 5 times tables are mastered, it is possible to understand forms of money. Understanding the forms of money based on 5x tables is elaborative and once the forms of money are understood, mastering money concepts comes very quickly and is easier and more pleasant than learning times tables but it could not be done without the rote learning of times tables early on.

Storage, of course, means that information has been received and kept in the brain. The problem with storage is that if the information cannot be retrieved, it cannot be used and might as well be lost, so the ability to recall or retrieve information is very important. Short term memory is quickly lost and never to be retrieved. Long term memory is kept and retrieved. In order to learn and master knowledge and skills, the information must be in long term memory and it must be accessible. Memory is created and strengthened by moving short term memory to long term memory.

There are two ways to convert short term memory to long term memory. The two ways are: rote learning or repetition and understanding. Rote learning or repetition is mechanical and repetitious and understanding is not required in order to save the information. Additionally, understanding requires comprehending the relationships between different facts and having the ability to arrive at conclusions or understanding.

The understanding form of memory would not be possible without some form of rote or repetition to begin with in order to have some data as a starting point. A good example is vocabulary. Vocabulary is learned by repetition or rote. Without understanding the words, the information delivered with language is useless. Learning by repetition is necessary to begin but learning by understanding must follow to acquire any mastery or ability.

Improving memory improves learning ability and increases capability. Once mastery of basic information in any area is mastered by repetition, it is possible to learn by understanding because more complex concepts can be grasped. In any situation and on any level it is easier to adapt and grow intellectually when memory is strong. Repetition is permanent improvement for long term memory and permits the intellectual growth to allow learning by understanding and engagement.

Once data is in place in long term memory, it needs to be remembered, or retrieved in order to be useful. There are practices that can be put into use to help retrieve memories or recall information that is needed:

1. Read, or study topics that are relevant to the memories that needs to be retrieved. Read or study regularly as opposed to many logging hours at one time.

2. Write down information that may be relevant or connected to the information that needs to be retrieved. This may trigger a memory.

3. Sing a song, or talk about things that are connected to the memory.

4. Relate or learn about information that is similar to what needs to be remembered.

5. Talk to someone about details of the memory that can be recalled if the actual memory cannot be retrieved.

7. Perform physical activity.

Lifelong learning is the key to strong memory that endures. In is not possible to escape repetition in order to learn further by understanding. In spite of the tedium and monotony of repetition, it is the gateway to higher level learning, competence and enjoyment. In learning any new information, repetition is the beginning of understanding. Repeated information is the first information to stay in long term memory and permit learning to occur at a higher and more rewarding level.

CHAPTER 6- THE IMPORTANCE OF BREATHING FOR MEMORY IMPROVEMENT

Breathing in oxygen is the foundation for which we are able to live our daily lives. Without oxygen we wouldn't live much longer than ten minutes. Our brains use the most oxygen than any other organ in our body and that is why it is very important to pay attention to oxygen intake when improving our memory.

When we take deep breaths in we get enough oxygen for our brains to function properly and for our body to remain healthy. Therefore in order to keep our memories sharp we have to maintain an adequate intake of oxygen every second of everyday in our lives. Without proper oxygen intake our brains will cease functioning properly and hence hinder our ability to remember what our tasks are. Another major concern of inadequate oxygen intake is the over-intake of carbon dioxide.

Carbon dioxide is a poisonous gas to humans and must be breathed out in proper amounts. When we hold in too much carbon dioxide we slowly kill our brain cells and thus kill our memory. Improper breathing such as quick breaths forces the body to contain large amounts of carbon dioxide. In order to maintain good memory we must breathe properly at all times. Not breathing properly inflicts great damage onto our brains and may make us feel dizzy or faint. Proper breathing is easily learned however takes a lot of practice to maintain.

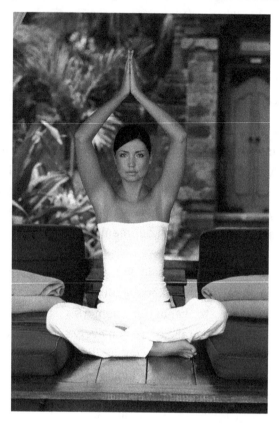

For proper breathing inhale slowly for 8 seconds, hold your breath for 4 seconds then exhale for another 8 seconds. Practice this every day starting with a 15 minute session and gradually advancing to longer periods of time. Proper inhaling should be done through the nose and exhaled through the mouth. Proper breathing also improves quality of sleep. The main reasons for humans losing the basic breathing technique are stress and anxiety.

Dealing with stress forces us to work faster and hence breathe more quickly. Anger also makes breath very fast and violently and messes with our normal cognition. Anxiety puts us in a state of fleeing in fear of our well-being and thus forces our breathing to become rapid. All these different stresses disturb the correct process of breathing and make us lose memory along with rational thinking. One great method some people use to improve their breathing is meditation.

Yogis in India perform meditation to help clear their mind and increase productive breathing. They sit in an upright position with their legs crossed (though crossing legs is optional) and hum for long periods of time. They also close one nostril and breath in deeply through the other nostril. After they breathe in they close the other nostril and slowly breathe out. These daily practices improve their memory as well as their overall health. These yogis are world-renowned for their knowledge of self-improvement so it would be wise to listen to them!

Whenever you are at work, home, a party, or anywhere that gives you the feeling of stress or anxiety you should remember the basic breathing pattern in order to calm down and allow your body to operate normally. If our body does not operate normally we cannot perform any tasks to our fullest potential. People who consciously remember to breath properly during exams and other stressful situations normally perform much better than those who underestimate the basic importance of proper breathing; hence those who breathe deeply and slowly are able to remember much more information needed for their daily tasks due to their brain working to the fullest extent.

Most people still underestimate the importance of basic necessities such as breathing due to taking the act for granted from birth. We believe may believe since we are still alive from the beginning of our lives that we know how to properly breath while those with much smaller egos pay attention to everything they have and thus breath in the most comfortable and natural way possible.

Most people believe the only important subjects to focus on are those that modern society enforce upon us with it "importance"; such as our careers, family lives, and financial well beings that we are to only focus on the perfections of what modern society asks of us while neglecting our basic functions of what makes us live our lives in true harmony. How can we remember our children's birthdays without a fully-functioning brain? How can we remember our spouse's anniversary's without a healthy memory?

Most people become so consumed with work and dealing with people that they take their basic bodily principles for granted. One must understand that it is okay to take 15 minutes or more a day to relax and focus on their breathing. Only with proper breathing can they remember everything they need to accomplish from their work life to their social life. Remembering birthdays, anniversaries and everything of the sort requires good memory and thus proper breathing. An anxious man is a man that will fail.

When we neglect proper breathing our respiratory muscles (located around the lungs) become weak. When we hurt our respiratory muscles we make it harder to breathe out and breathe in. Therefore before we try to remember anything we must exercise our larynx (diaphragm). If you cannot breathe deeply and slowly from your nose to your mouth than consider using Bellows breathing which is breathing quickly using only your nose. Although not as beneficial to your body as the proper breathing technique, Bellows breathing will lower stress levels and increase the production of the hormone epinephrine which is crucial to memory.

People have been practicing various breathing techniques through methods such as yoga and meditation for hundreds of years and thus have been able to remember all their basic responsibilities whether they included family or business matters. Stress is one of the number 1 killers of human beings and it begins with destroying our breathing patterns. If we can't remember what we're supposed to do then how can we live our daily lives to the fullest?

CHAPTER 7- WHY IT IS IMPORTANT TO VARY THE ROUTINES FOR MEMORY IMPROVEMENT EXERCISES

Exercises for improving memory abilities center on optimally stimulating many regions within the brain. When the brain obtains new information, it goes through a detailed process, ultimately sorting and storing the new data in the long-term and short-term memory centers of the brain. By taking in and storing recently learned information or tasks, we stimulate regions housed within the vast network of the brain. Although memory improvement exercises are an excellent tool for maintaining optimum brain function, is important to vary these exercise routines.

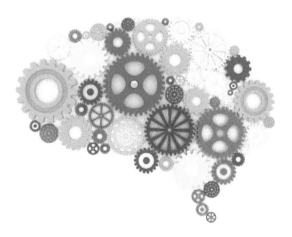

The concept behind memory exercises is similar to a physical workout. During a physical workout routine, each exercise focuses on one particular muscle within the body. An individual seeking to strengthen arm muscles may lift weights with steady repetitions. However, in order to reach optimal health throughout the entire body, a workout schedule should include exercises specifically focused on each muscle group for attaining overall peak condition.

These same concepts apply when exercising the brain as well. Varying your memory improvement exercises ensures each region within the detailed network receives healthy stimulation.

Depending on the type of information we take in also stipulates which regions the brain uses when processing, filtering and storing the new data. The first step toward the memory process triggers our sensory abilities i.e. smell, sound, taste. For example, when introduced to a new flower, our brains register the aroma, the color and texture of the plant.

After triggering the sensory function, the brain then decides whether to store this new information into short-term or long-term memory sectors. For this to occur, nerve cells begin to stimulate through an electrical charge or pulse. This stimulated action sends a message to our neurotransmitters, which then link cells together. As more links connect, the cells become stronger, the same way our muscles become stronger through a variety of physical exercise.

During the intake of information, our brains conduct an elaborate series of duties while exercising many areas within this vast network. When performing memory-improving concepts, a variety of regimens allows an individual to stimulate specific brain functions by always introducing new concepts. Whenever an individual learns and takes in new data, the brain continually rewires and sorts previously stored information while making room for new memories. Consistently changing a memory-improving task activates and stimulates cell connections, sensory receptors and neurotransmitter functions.

Within our brain lies the cerebral cortex, which consists of four distinct lobes and is responsible for overall processing of information. Each lobe's function is unique. The medial temporal lobe regulates our long and short-term memory while our frontal lobe handles decision-making. Our parietal lobe stimulates and processes data through navigational tasks and our occipital lobe works through the process of sight. Each of these lobes stimulates deeper regions within the cerebral cortex such as the ability for retrieving stored information. Because each area performs a specific task, it is important to introduce a variety of exercises for affecting multiple layers of the cerebral cortex.

If one area of the brain fails to receive stimulation or becomes dormant due to lack of activity, over time the nerve cells begin to shut down. This is the primary reason why a vast array of specific memory-improving tasks and exercises are vital for achieving and maintaining healthy brain function as we age. Throughout an average lifetime, introducing new learning concepts keeps every area active and healthy.

A helpful tip to remember when performing a daily memory-improving routine is to constantly introduce new challenges. Brain inactivity occurs when a learned task becomes repetitive. Over time, we no longer trigger the learning sections of the brain; the activity no longer categorizes as learned rather becoming habitual. This means some cells no longer activate as they would when absorbing new data, becoming dormant from lack of use. Variety is the key to an optimal memory-improving program.

By regularly introducing a new thinking task, brain cell formation constantly occurs. Learning new concepts produces new cell growth. Therefore, constructing memory-improving schedules around several types of exercises stimulates each region. With the advancement of technology comes a huge resource of computerized programs geared specifically toward healthy brain cell formation while avoiding redundancy. The internet offers games specializing in memory function tasks rotated on a consistent basis. Other on-line concepts utilize the brains hand-eye coordination centers while some offer intricate mathematical problems, benefiting our learning centers. Memory-improvement exercises also include regimens where participation requires the use of both hands. By incorporating use of our non-dominant hand, our brain inadvertently applies a new task that requires extensive concentration.

Brain exercise programs require constant change for challenging the numerous functions within the entire network and any routine should cover all areas of brain functioning. This process improves concentration levels and mental clarity while boosting memory capabilities as well. Also helpful, implementing activities that require using more than one sense at the same time offers a beneficial avenue toward proper mental exercise. For example, the simple act of listening to your favorite music while performing household tasks generates the function of several senses at once. Performing a repetitive action such as brushing your hair with your non-dominant hand triggers multiple-sensory stimulation.

By varying routines within a daily memory-improvement schedule, individuals guarantee each area receives optimal stimulation on a consistent basis. Applying ever-changing task rotation aids in boosting brainpower abilities and encourages the creation of new neurons, which serve as the basis for overall brain function. Repetitive tasks performed over a length of time become expected. Once our brain reaches a repetitive stage, receptors not regularly in use begin shutting down. When these receptors remain dormant, they can stagnate, ultimately losing the ability for functioning again.

While educated throughout the primary school years, the brain receives constant overall stimulation as the volume of data continues to change. During this period, the brain functions at peak healthy levels. Once our primary education ends, receiving varied stimuli becomes paramount toward a healthy brain. Adopting

Jason Scotts

varying levels within any memory-improvement exercise regimen is necessary for achieving recall and memory capabilities.

ABOUT THE AUTHOR

Raised in a home where learning was encouraged Jason Scotts was exposed to quite a number of things form an early age. As he matured he was exposed to even more things until it came to a point where he was able to follow up on his own interests. As such he developed an interest in memory improvement among other things.

Jason was interested in learning everything that he could about improving memory as he was finding that he was challenged with remembering certain things. He did the necessary research and found quite a few ideas that he tried; some worked well and some not so well.

This led him to start working on another book that would just highlight all the ones that he found worked for him and his friends that he had asked to try it as well. The greatest thing is that these methods would have shown some level of success in just a month.

Printed in the USA
CPSIA information can be obtained
at www.ICGtesting.com
LVHW082129280124
770104LV00055B/1318

9 781628 847284